Healing Herbs

How To Make Money Growing Herbs

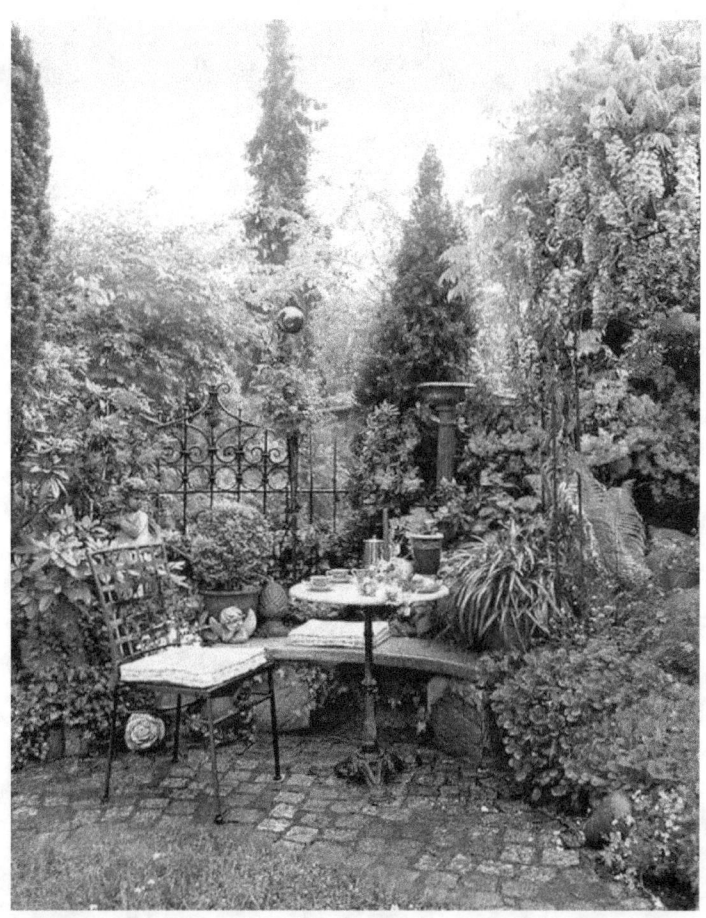

Table of content

Introduction

I wish to thank and congratulate you for downloading *"Healing Herbs: How to Make Money Growing Herbs."* You will have a great time reading through this book and learning how to pick and choose the right herbs for you to add to your personal herb garden. If you are having any concerns on whether you can become a 'green thumb' in herb gardening then you can put your mind at ease when you read chapter 1. In that chapter I have compiled a list of herbs and the best methods to propagate them, and the best environments for them to thrive in. If you are planning on making money from your herbal garden you first must learn how to setup a thriving healthy herb garden. We will go through the steps so that by the end of this book you will be prepared to setup and start making money on your healing herbs.

You are soon going to discover that owning a herb garden is something that is going to bring you a sense of satisfaction and have a very therapeutic effect on you. Maintaining your herb garden is something that you should look upon as a luxury not a burden. Once you begin to read further and further into this book you will understand what I mean when I say it is a wonderfully relaxing hobby to get into or a fun source of income. Now it is time to begin working on that 'green thumb' of yours starting with chapter 1—enjoy your journey towards happy gardening and getting into the green with profits from your healing herbs!

Chapter 1. Different Types of Herbs

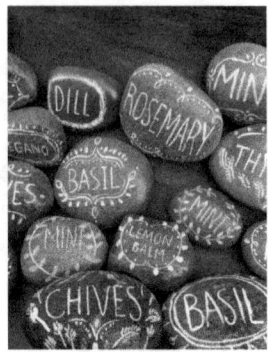

The answer to why you should grow a herb garden will lie in what kinds of herbs that you wish to grow within your herb garden. Are you leaning more towards growing medicinal herbs or culinary or perhaps a bit of both? Before you begin digging and sorting out soil, you need to sit down and decide what kinds of herbs you want to include in your herb garden. Make a list of herbs that are your favorite choices of herbs that you want to grow in your herb garden. If you are planning to grow them for profit you will of course have to decide the best herbs for you to grow in order for you to make money from them.

If you are growing culinary herbs are you going to want herbs that you can dry and some that you can have fresh? Perhaps you have a plan of making some flavored oils and vinegars to give as gifts to loved ones or sell at a local farmers market? Maybe you have recently discovered some of the wonderful health benefits that herbs offer and you are interested in growing herbs to make infusions, teas and pastes to help you and your loved ones minor health conditions or sell to others?

It is important to know what plants that you want to focus on growing. If you are more interested in growing herbs for culinary reasons then you should focus on the herbs that will help add much flavor to your meals or your customers meals. You will also have to decide on how big of a garden you are planning on having. This will of course help decide how many plants you will be able to grow in it. I would suggest as a beginner you should start at with a fairly small garden then once you become more comfortable with gardening you can expand. You may want to start off with container gardening, these can be used indoors and outdoors. It is important that you are aware of the amount of space that you have to use for your herbal garden. However I will presume that you have a fairly large herbal garden and are now thinking of ways that you can perhaps make an income from your herbs. Let us first take a look at the different kinds of herbs that you might be have an interest in growing.

Culinary herbs. Many people use the culinary herbs most often in adding flavor to their meals. People that have added fresh herbs to their meals know how much they can benefit the flavor of a meal. How wonderful is spaghetti that has fresh basil sprinkled on top of it, and fresh oregano, or how adding some fresh chopped chives to the top of your baked potato and sour cream—yes I can taste that yummy flavor now!

Culinary herbs are often referred to as sweet herbs—these can be annual, biennial, perennial plants that have tender roots or have ripe seeds. This class of herb also offers an aromatic flavor—they smell so good and they taste great! One common herb that has been used in many households in the kitchen is parsley.

Aromatic herbs. This type of herbs is usually used to add into products and are not used very often in a culinary capacity. They are instead used often in products such as toilet water, perfumes, amongst other items that are full of fragrance. You may want to grow aromatic herbs in your garden to make poultices to sell to others made of herbs such as lavender.

Ornamental herbs. You may want to grow some herbs that will add vitality to your environment and brighten it up. There are many herbs that have lovely bright flowers that would enhance any where you chose to display them. This type of herbs are mainly for decorative purposes, but there are those that will overlap into other categories of herbs such as culinary and medicinal. You may just decide never to harvest these plants but rather keep them as a decorative plant in your garden.

Valerian would be a good choice in this type of herb as they are also a very valuable medicinal herb—this would be what I would call the perfect choice, also keep in mind other herbs that are also good choices such as lavender, and even chives. The Dittany of Crete is another perfect example of the ornamental herb. It is actually a type of Oregano. It forms a low mound producing lovely fine leaves with silvery hairs. This plant was not meant to add flavor to meals—it was created to appeal to the eye not the stomach!

Medicinal Herbs. The medicinal herbs are probably the most prized of all types of herbs, especially for our ancestors that depended on them so very much to get them through illnesses. There was a point in our human history when almost every family had someone in their family tree that was a herbalist or amateur herbalist. The use of herbal medicine is indeed the oldest form of health care or treatment to humans. Cultures from all over the world used plants to treat ailments and still do today. Many of the best and most effective prescription drugs of today began as herbs.

If you are planning on growing medicinal herbs to perhaps sell to make money you need to know exactly what kinds of herbs are geared to treat what ailments. The herb Echinea was widely used before the discovery of antibiotics. It is making a comeback because it has an outstanding ability to help to boost the immune system.

Often today people will take this herb in a capsule in order to fend off colds or flu. Echinacea is one of the easiest medicinal herbs to grow, and also looks very appealing to the eye. It has a flower that is similar to the structure of a daisy. They have an extended period of blooming so they make a nice addition to your garden. This plant will begin to bloom in spring and will continue to bloom until the fall months. It is a very hardy plant, it can survive hot dry summers. Now you have a better idea of types of herbs in the next chapter we will take a closer look at individual top ten culinary and medicinal herbs.

Chapter 2. Top 10 Culinary and Medicinal Herbs

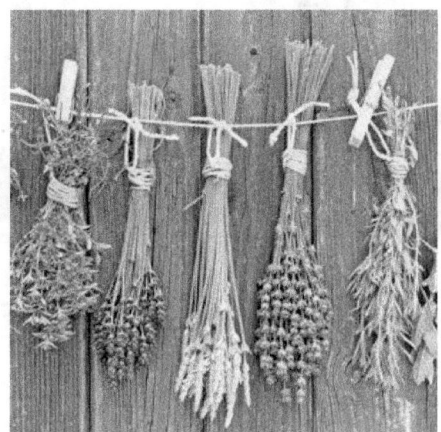

In this chapter we are going to have a look at the top ten culinary and medicinal herbs. This will help to give you a better idea of what kinds of herbs you will decide to grow.

Top Ten Culinary Herbs:

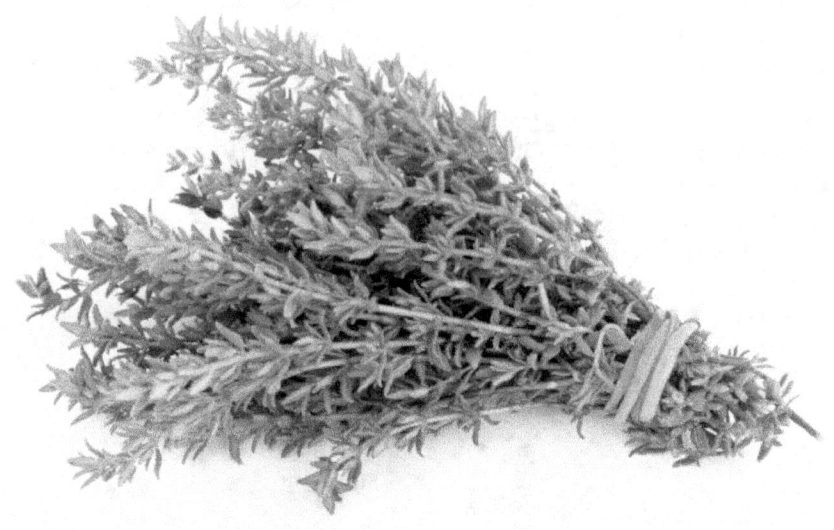

1. Thyme—this herb is a great herb to add to your herbal garden. It really works well as a great seasoning for meat. Rub it on beef, veal, lamb, pork before you put it in the oven. You can also add it to eggs, veggie and cheese dishes. Try it with fish and poultry as well. It is also a popular seasoning for stews, soups, stuffing as well as in rice. Some people use it to make thyme tea with adding in a sprig of mint and rosemary. This herb you can start from seeds in mid-spring in shallow rows for the seeds, planting the seeds about one foot apart. You may also choose to start growing them from seedlings.

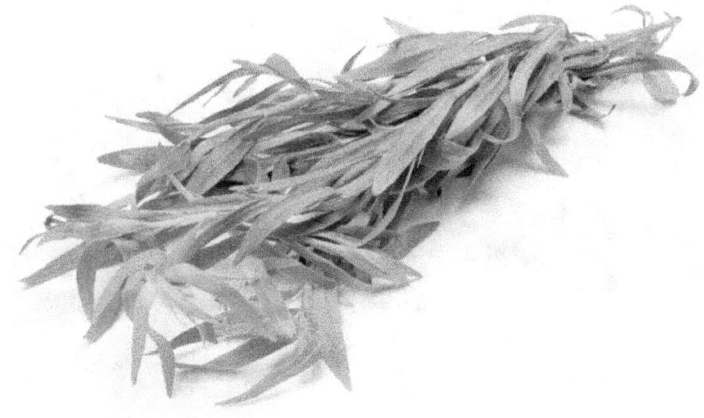

2. Tarragon—this herb makes a wonderful flavoring for vinegar. Grow your own tarragon and add it to your vinegar yourself. Try adding to soups, stews, and salads. Use in egg dishes or cheese dishes.

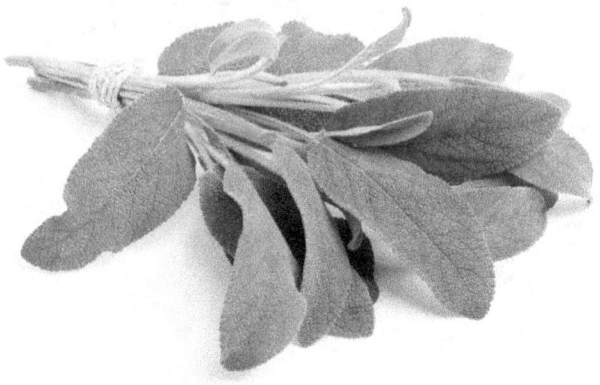

3. Sage—this herb can work wonders in adding to the flavor of your culinary dishes. It works great in sweet sausage, or chicken and turkey stuffing. Many cooks love to use sage with lamb and pork dishes as well. It is often used in different cheese dishes and omelets. You can grow this plant easily from seed, plant in early spring. You may also choose to buy seedlings from nursery and plant about a foot apart.

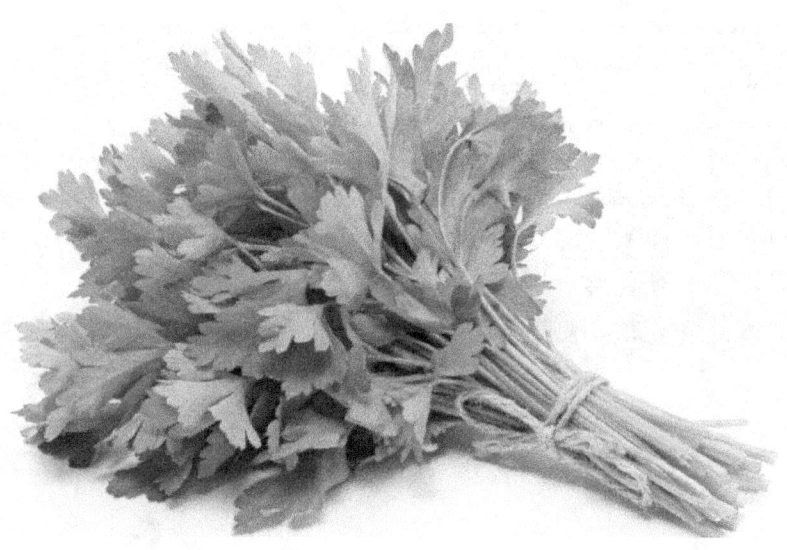

4. Parsley—this is a herb that many people use in their daily meals all around the world. It is very popular in soups, casseroles, salads and makes a great garnish for many dishes. Plant seeds in mid-spring. Before you plant the seeds soak them overnight in water.

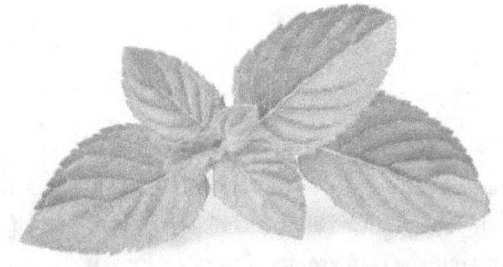

5. Mint—this is an essential herb, this is a herb that will work well in a culinary herb garden or a medicinal, or a little bit of both is what I personally choose to grow. You can enjoy some mint leaves in a cup of tea or use them to add some flavor to cold drinks or to be used for garnish. It is the favored spice to use when preparing lamb. Sprinkle some dry or fresh leaves over the meat just before you cook it. You should plant your mint in the autumn or spring. You will have the best results if you start with seedlings. Make sure that you plant them two inches deep and about a foot apart.

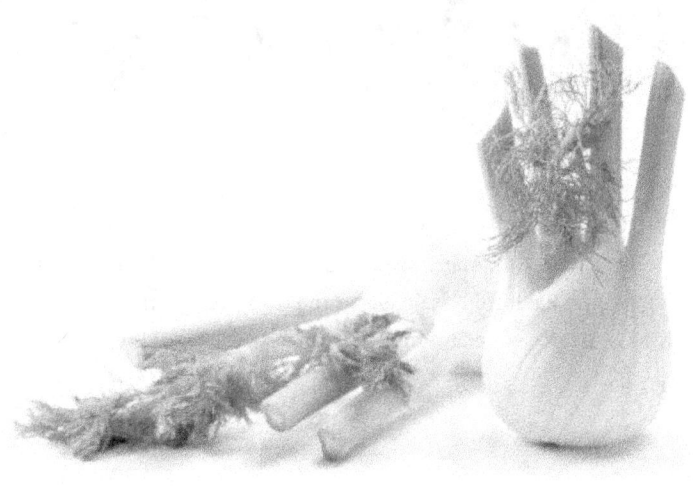

6. Fennel—this is a herb you should try the next time that you prepare fish, you can create a wonderful tasting sauce using it. It also works wonders with pork and veal. Many people enjoy using it in making soups and salads. The seeds have a bit of a sharp flavor and the leaves are sweet. Plant your seeds in groups of three or four at around mid-spring. Dig a hole about one quarter of an inch deep. Place the seeds about a foot apart. You will have to thin them when they begin to grow into seedlings.

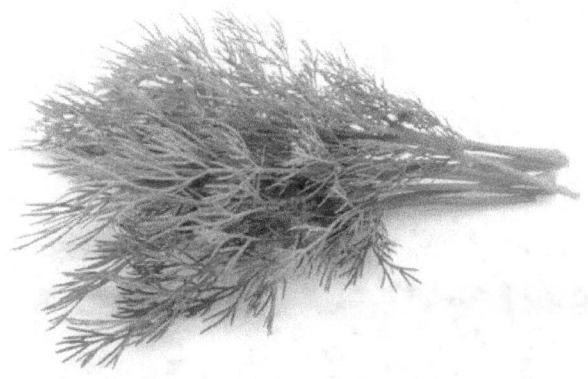

7. Dill—this is a herb that you can use the seeds and the leaves. Both the dill leaves and seeds have a bit of a bitter taste to them. Whether you decide to use dill fresh or dried it will add flavor to your meat, poultry and fish dishes. You can also add it to soups and salads. Many people enjoy using the leaves in omelets and potatoes. You can also sprinkle some on cucumbers being used as a sandwich filling. It is another easy plant that you can grow from seed in early spring. Make a whole about one quarter of an inch deep, and have about ten inches between your seeds. Once your seedlings appear you will need to thin them out.

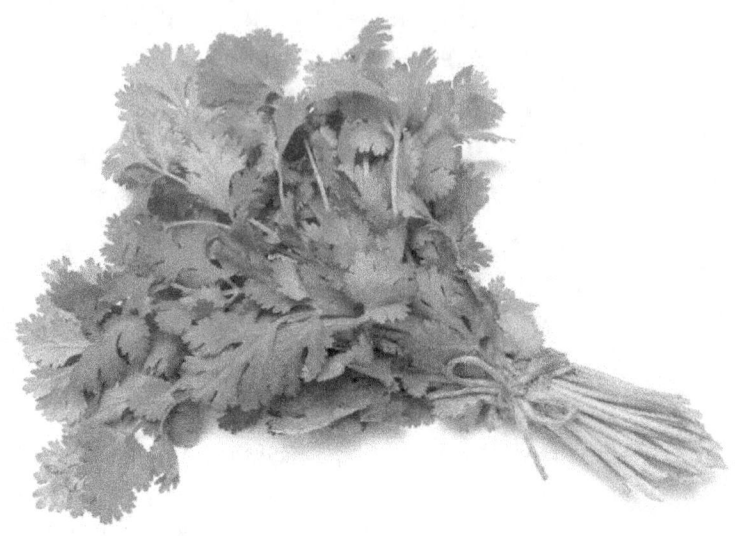

8. Coriander—this is a herb that is so versatile that different parts of this plant are known as different herbs. You can grind the seeds to use in pork, ham or veal. You can use the leaves in Asian or Indian dishes this is called cilantro. You can also use the roots of coriander. You can freeze the parts of the plant that you are not going to use right away. Enjoy using them to flavor soups, chop up the roots and serve them with avocados. Coriander is easy to grow from seed, sow the seed in early spring. Digging a hole about one quarter of an inch deep. Plant the seeds about a foot apart in a row.

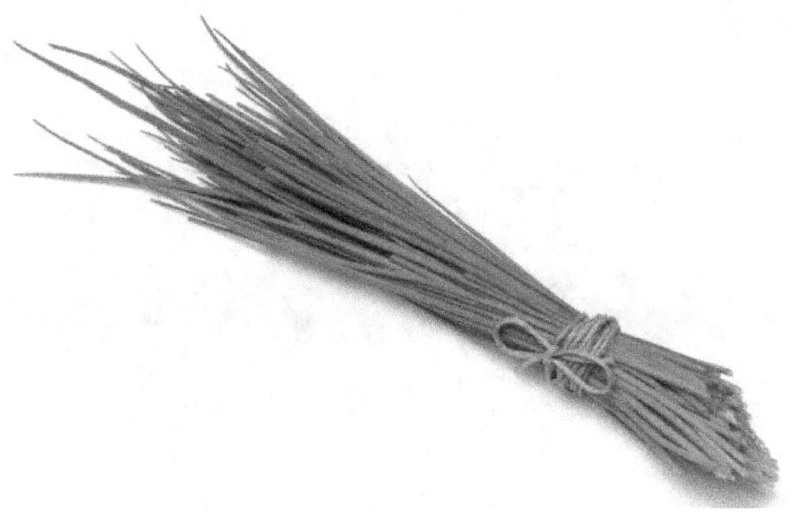

9. Chives—this is a herb that is wonderful with a dollop of sour cream on a baked potato. Chives have a kind of onion-like taste to them. They are a great addition to salads, cream cheese, sandwich spreads, egg and cheese dishes and sauces. Try some chives in your mashed potatoes as well as your baked potato. Start with seedlings and plant in early spring. Give the plants plenty of room about a foot apart from each other.

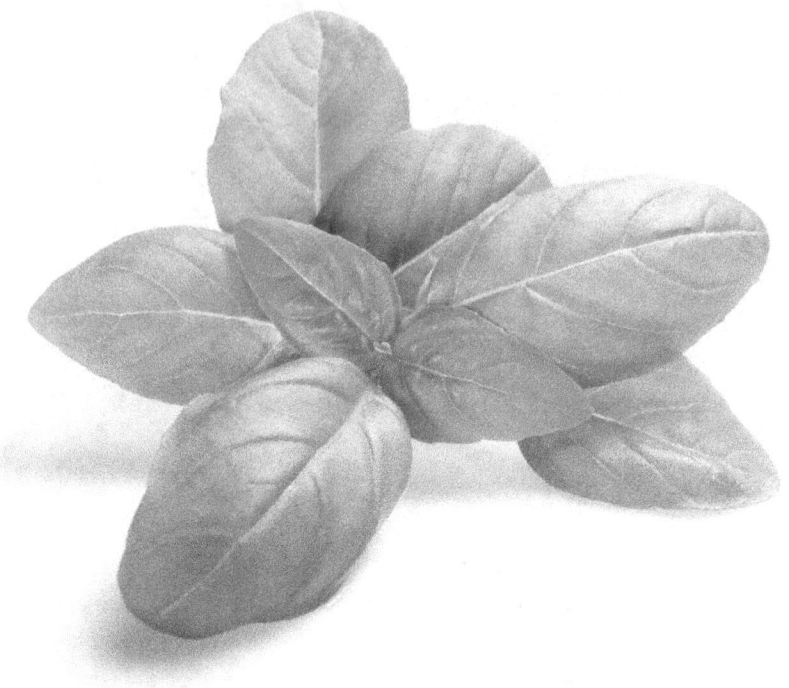

10. Basil—this herb works when you are preparing a pesto. It leaves a lovely spicy flavor. You only need a small amount of this herb to add flavor to your dishes. It works great in soups, salads and sauces. In works very well in tomato dishes. Use it to enhance the flavor of your meat, fish and poultry. Add it to your nice big omelet in the morning. Start growing basil seedling in early spring, preferably in a greenhouse setting, or on a sunny window sill.

Top 10 Medicinal Herbs:

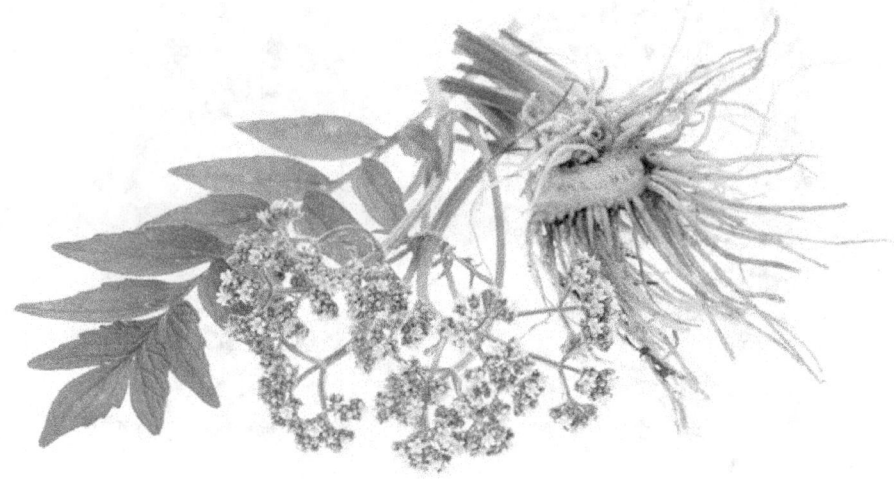

1. Valerian—this is a plant that you should truly consider for your herbal garden. The first one or two years you will not find flowers on this plant nor will they smell especially good. But if you want to become serious in your herbalism then you should add this plant to your herb garden. It is a versatile herb it has been used throughout history to treat various ailments. It is said to be a great natural treatment for anxiety, restlessness or tension. It is also good in treating a variety of stomach ailments such as cramps and digestive issues. Just because it may lack in flowers it has plenty of uses. Another great plus with this plant is it can grow just about anywhere! If you have a section of your garden that is rather moist try placing your Valerian plants there.

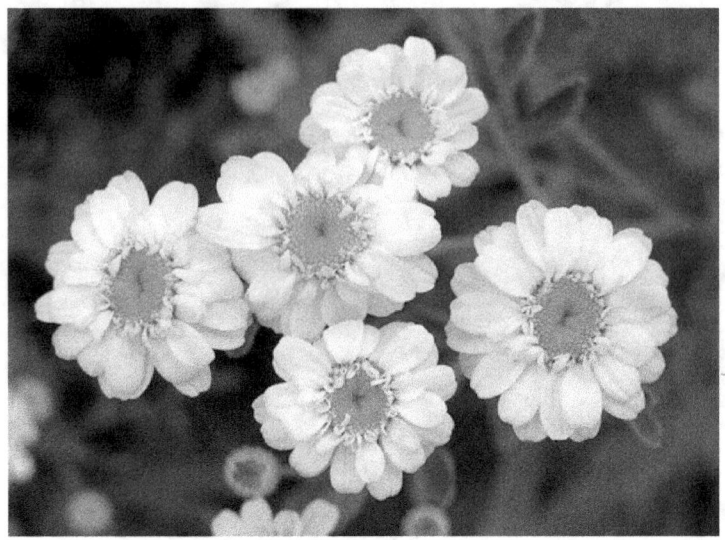

2. Feverfew—this may not be a name that you are familiar with, but the flower I am sure you will be. Feverfew, it has been known for centuries as a natural cure for migraine headaches, the flower of this herb resembles the daisy. It has white petals and yellow center with green serrated leaves. These flowers can grow to be about two feet tall. Many people have used this plant to help treat their arthritis and rheumatism. It blooms almost all summer long. Feverfew is not a fussy plant and it grows in most types of soil. It is a great plant to place between stones of pavers in your garden. You will probably have no problem growing this plant from seed.

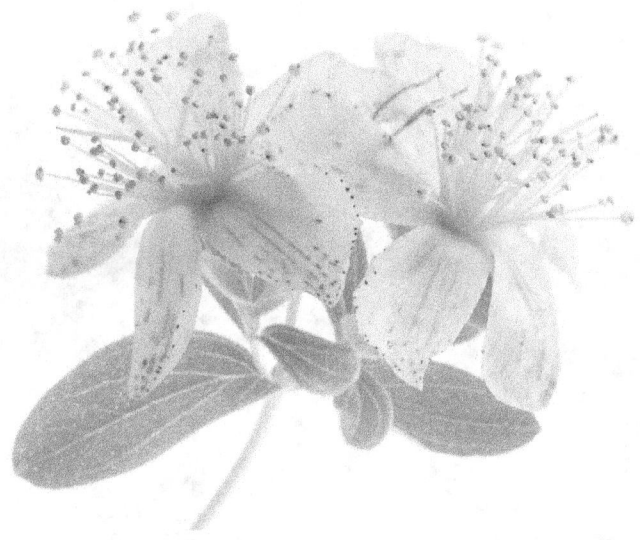

3. St. John's Wort—this herb is not native to the United States, but you can find it today growing along the roadside in many regions where the weather conditions are mild. It blooms from late May through to September, depending on the climate you are growing it in. The name comes from the timing of its flowering. It was believed that the flower bloomed on St. John the Baptist's birthday.

I am sure you are aware of this herb as a healing herb. It has gotten close scrutiny from the medical community. It is best used in treating depression. You should have no problem starting it from seed. It will grow just about anywhere, it will grow well in full to partial sun and in shade. It will thrive in moist light soils.

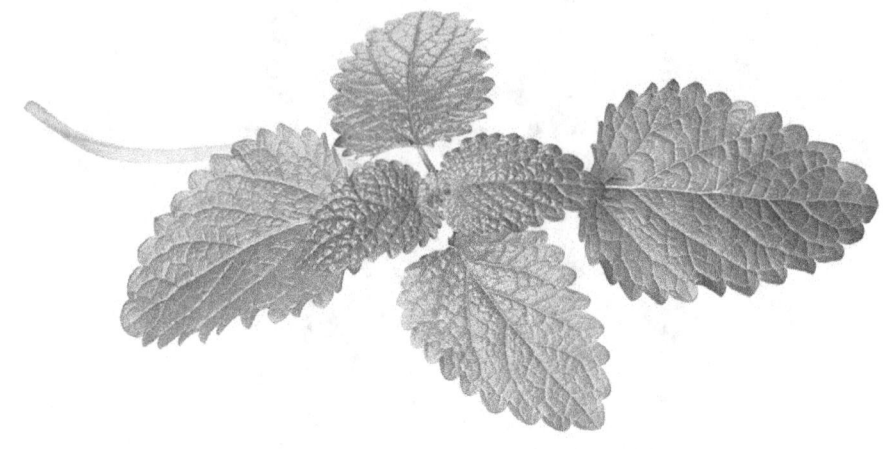

4. Lemon Balm—this is a herb that is a basic staple of every healing herb garden. It was originally native to Europe, lemon balm is now found everywhere around the planet. It has similar medicinal traits as mint. It will help with digestive system issues and is also used in the relieving digestive pain. People that have anxiety or nervousness or insomnia use this plant with much success. The most common way people use this herb is to steep the leaves and prepare a tea. It is part of the mint family and will grow to be about one foot in height. It has the wonderful aroma and taste of lemon. It is easy to grow outside. It will grow in clumps and will spread. The stems of the plant will die off in winter, but no need to worry they will shoot up in the spring once again. You can also try growing lemon balm from stem cuttings or from seed. Plant them about one foot apart.

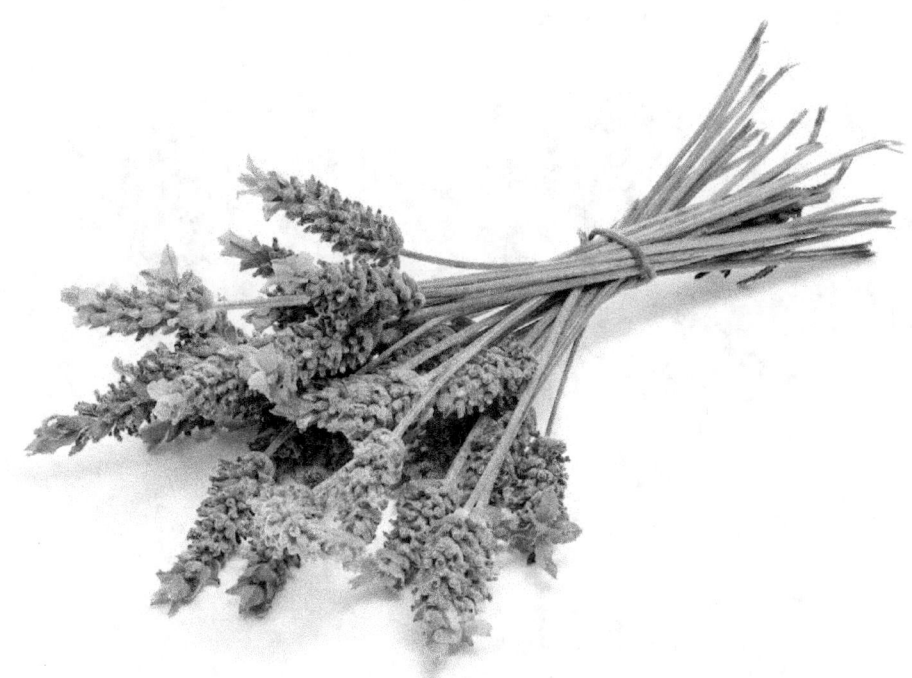

5. **Lavender**—this is a herb that no healing garden should be without. Lavender is wonderful in healing pain much like Echinacea is to boosting the immune system— indispensable! There is many health benefits connected to Lavender. It has a great help in relieving pain and helping us to relax. Lavender works great in relieving anxiety. It is often used to help cure insomnia and as a muscle relaxant. It is also suspected of helping support healthy blood pressure levels. The plant has a lovely bluish-grey needle-like foliage topped with lovely violet-blue flowers. The long-blooming flowers are going to give you visual pleasure all throughout the growing season. It is a drought-tolerant plant, making it very easy to care for. Keep your plant in a well-drained area.

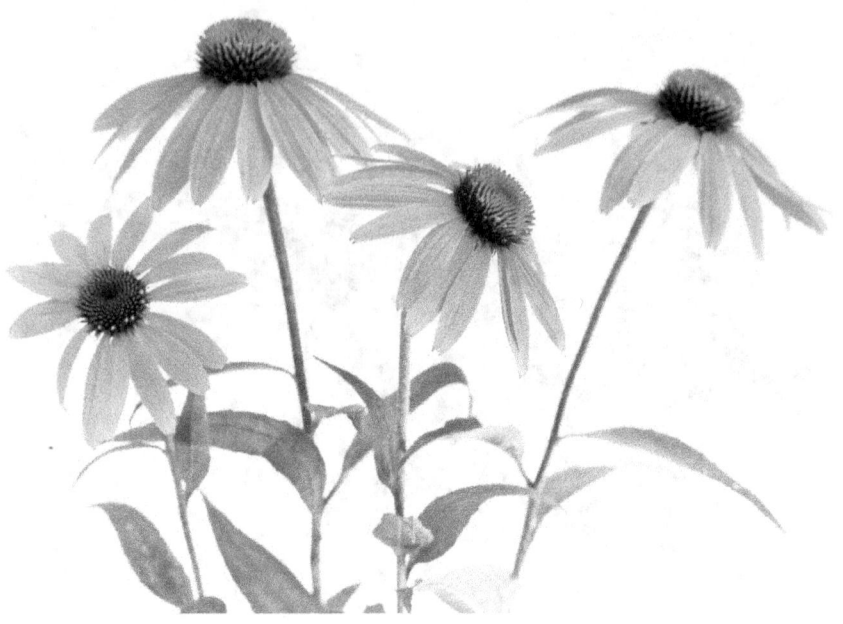

6. Echinacea—this would certainly be a great addition to your healing garden. This plant has wonderful properties. It is a great and powerful booster for your immune system. Many people take this herb in a capsule form to avoid catching the flu or cold during the cold winter months. It has a wonderful large purple flower it is also referred to as the purple cone flower. It comes in three varieties: Echinacea angustifolia, Echinacea pallid, and Echinacea pupuea. All three varieties have similar medicinal effects.

Echinacea is also used in treating many respiratory infections by many herbalists. It is very easy to grow and is very tolerant of dry conditions. You should be able to grow it from seed no problem. Plant the seeds in the spring once the soil has reached about 70° Fahrenheit. Within 10-20 days you should see the seeds sprouting. Cover the tops of them with some more soil. Thin the plants when they are seedlings to about one foot apart. The plant prefers to have shade over full sun. You may want to test your soils pH balance before you plant your seeds. This plant prefers neutral soil which will read to be between six to eight. The

Echinacea plant will bloom from June to October and it will attract the butterflies to your garden. It is wonderful when you go out to your garden and see the butterflies floating and hovering about the Echinacea in your garden.

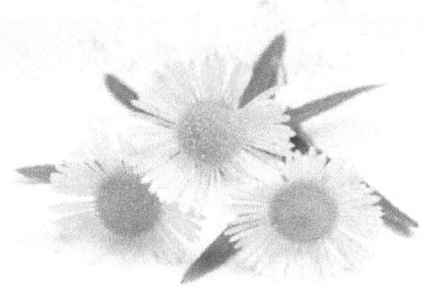

7. Chamomile—this is one of the best known healing herbs. It is a popular choice of tea. It is a good choice of tea to have before you go to sleep or when you are feeling that your nerves are shot or are agitated. It has calming effects on humans. It has been also discovered that it may also help to boost your immune system, making you more resistant to colds and flu. You can begin to grow this herb and make your very own tea from scratch. It is easy to grow from seed and it does well in average soil and loves to be in the full sun. Plant your seeds in early spring. Once your seedlings grow thin them out to be about one foot apart. When you harvest this plant wait until the flowers are at peak bloom. You can use this plant for remedies either fresh or dried. To dry the flowers that is easy. You just have to spread them out in a cool and well-ventilated place. Use the flowers to brew yourself some nice relaxing tea. You can also mix the flowers with other kinds of tea and make your own unique blend. You can serve it as an ice tea or hot or even mix it into a punch mixture.

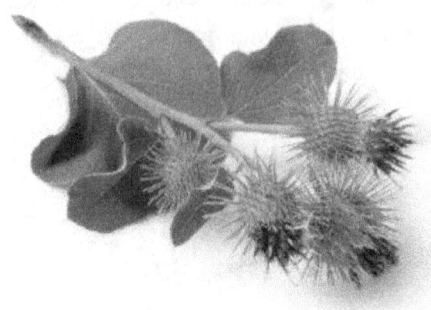

8. Burdock—this is a herb that you will probably not find in a lot of gardens, but adding it to your garden will make your garden that much more distinctive. Some refer to this herb as gobo. Drinking Burdock tea will help with gastrointestinal tract issues and is also used to boost one's appetite. It has also been used to help restore liver function with herbalists. Burdock can be found growing freely in many areas. Most people grow it from seed, planting it in early spring—the earlier the better. Cover the seeds with about one quarter of an inch of soil. When you plant the seeds make sure that the soil is moist. You should notice the sprouts in about seven days. Take the seedlings and thin them out until they are about three inches apart. The plant prefers the full sun, but it can tolerate some shade. It prefers a well-drained soil, and free of rocks and stones.

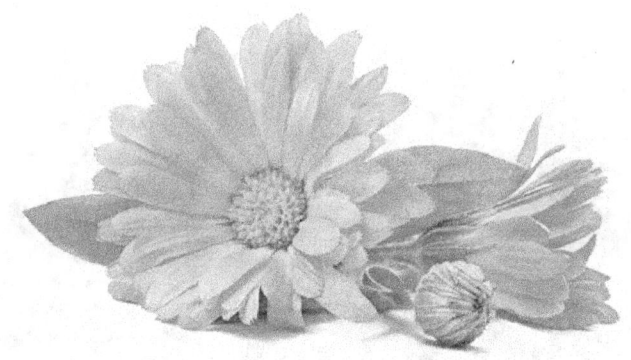

9. Calendula—this plant has lovely bright flowers, and is a great plant to add to your healer's garden. Many people often will call it a marigold, it is also called Calendula. It is one of the most versatile healing herbs. I have this plant in my own garden. It has a wonderful orange blossom, it can be used for a nice soothing skin wash, salve or a tea. The flower itself is also edible. Garnish your next salad with some Calendula petals. It is often used in salves for skin irritations such as diaper rash and other baby related items.

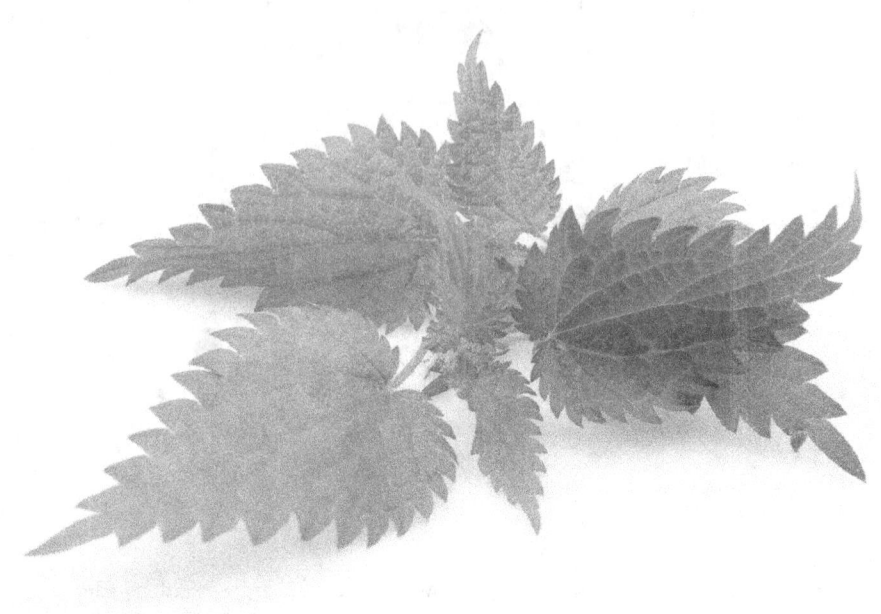

10. Nettles—this is a plant that is easy to grow, it is effective in helping to heal inflammation due to allergies, lupus and arthritis. It is also used as tonic to help alleviate the symptoms of anemia. This plant is rich in vitamin C and iron. Herbalists use the leaves and the roots of this plant for treating various symptoms. This plant is also full of many various antioxidants and flavonoids. Plant in early spring the seeds and thin them out to be one foot or so apart.

Chapter 3. Keeping Your Plants Healthy and Happy!

When you are planting or transplanting your herbs I would suggest adding a dash of compost or bone meal into the hole where you are placing the seedlings or seeds to help with drainage and to add some extra nutrients. As you begin to grow herbs you will soon realize that most herbs grow best in an alkaline soil, so you may want to add a tablespoon or so of agricultural lime. This is going to help the roots of your herbs to absorb the nutrients more efficiently. You mix it into the hole before you put in your herb plant. You can start herbs indoors and then transfer them later into outside garden once the weather is warm enough.

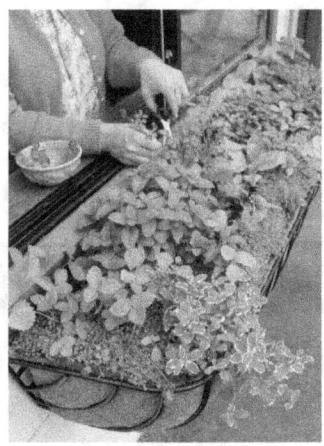

Some plants you may want to consider starting indoors are sorrel, catnip, chamomile, marjoram, oregano, basil, borage and thyme. Place the seeds in flats that are well-drained with airy soil with lots of organic matter. Borage and sorrel prefer to be in soil that is moist and rich. When your seedlings are about four inches tall and the weather is nice and warm you can now take them outside to plant in your outside garden. You should not take them outdoors until the overnight temperatures rise to a dependable 50° Fahrenheit or more. You will introduce them to the outdoors by first placing the flats outside in early morning. Leave them for several hours. You are dealing with delicate seedlings so do not take them out on really windy days. They are frail at this point and can break their stems easily. Don't allow the soil to dry out especially when first putting them outside.

Repeat this introduction process for about five or six days. Each day increase the amount of time that you leave the seedlings outside. If it is too hot or heavy rain do not put them out. After you have completed this process your seedlings should be climatized to the outdoors and ready to be planted in your outdoor garden. You may also choose to water them less and less before you plant them outside. Allow the soil to dry a little more each time you do this for about two weeks. Eventually you will only water them when they begin to droop, when they get to this point they are ready to be introduced to the outside garden.

Propagating your new plants. Once you have planted your herbs into your outside garden and they appear to be doing nicely you are ready to take the next step in propagating your new plants. There is three main methods to do this. You can create more plants by dividing the roots of the plant, by taking cuttings of the herbs in your gardens, or through a method called "healing-in' or layering.

Root division. This is an easy approach for you to create more plants. With a spade or shovel, work out the roots of from a densely growing herb. Take this grouping and separate the plants starting by the roots. Do this very carefully. Once you have separated them you can place one of them back into the original hole again. Take the other group and plant them where you would like them.

Creating herbs from cuttings. This approach is also pretty straight-forward to propagating herbs. In the spring or fall, take a long woody shoot from the plant of your choosing, cut this shoot from the plant. Cut the shoot at an angle close to the grand. Remove the leaves from the bottom of this cutting. Coat it with rooting powder and pot it in a light soil mix. Water it well.

Creating new herbs through the use of layering. You start by bending a long woody shoot and bury the middle of the stem under a few inches of soil. Hold it in place with a small rock. Within a month or so the healed-in stem develops its own root system. When it does you are then able to transplant it.

Chapter 4. Ways You Can Make Money with Your Healing Herbs

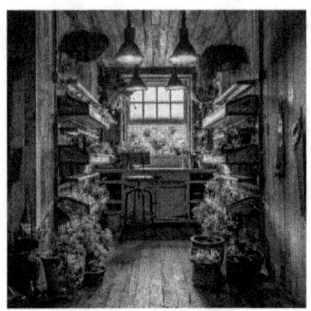

You could find that your attempts at making money from your herbs you actually end up sending you up and into a financial realm that you had no idea was possible. To start with perhaps you could use your garage as a place to setup up shop so to speak. You could get a bit creative and make your garage your herb shop. You could set it up with dried herbs, herbal preparations, seedlings for sale, and other herbal related products. You could dry or sell fresh herbs and seedlings.

You can certainly take the passion that you have for growing herbs and build it into a viable source of income for yourself. Just think how close it is for you to travel to work—it will literally be a hop, skip and a jump—no long commutes. You may want to consider starting small selling one or two seedling varieties perhaps and some dried herbs. From this you can build and expand your herbal selling empire. Use your passion for growing herbs to help finance any expansions you may be planning for your garden. You may only be interested in selling a few herbs here and there. Whether you choose to sell culinary or medicinal or both there is a market for both.

Taking the step into making a business out of your herbs. Below I have provided you with five ways that you can change this hobby into a business. In this economy there is more and more people looking for products that are organically grown and are locally produced.

Selling Seeds. You could start off your business by selling seeds and seedlings. This is one of the easiest ways to begin a business from your herbs. Decide if you are selling culinary or medicinal herbs. You must put yourself in the customer's shoes and decide what herbs most customers are likely interested in. Perhaps you want to offer herbs that are hard to find in your area—people will love to find out that you have special herbs they love but have trouble getting them in your area. You may choose basil as your culinary herb of choice and for medicinal you may choose Echinacea.

What to do to market yourself. You may feel that marketing yourself will be a big challenge. In reality it is really easy. Word of mouth is a great marketing tool. Tell your family friends of your business plans and get them to spread the word. You can also go around to local businesses and ask to put a flyer up at their store. Many grocery stores and restaurants are more than happy to do this for the locals. These are quick and inexpensive ways to let the public know about your herb business. You may also choose to place a classified ad in your local paper.

Take a day to set up your plants and seedlings at the local farmers market or flea market. These would be perfect venues. Even set up a little stand at the end of your drive to sell plants and seedlings from there at the roadside. You should get some business cards made up, some websites will offer you a free starter pack where you will only pay for the shipping and handling charges.

When to start. You are going to want to begin growing herbs you want to sell in the late winter and very early spring. Begin with two or so kinds of herbs. You want to keep them nice and healthy so they will look great when it is time to sell them. You want to offer you clients top quality seedlings and plants that are not too expensive.

You want your customers to remember you and the good quality plants you sold at a reasonable and affordable price. So these customers will continue to come back for more and more plants each season.

Selling dried herbs. There are many people that love herbs but have no desire to grow them. If you sell herbs that have been organically grown and tenderly dried with care—then you will expand your customer base by doing this. Many people love to buy fresh dried herbs that are organically grown locally. Sell your dried and fresh herbs right beside each other this is giving your customers more selection and options.

When you are selling your herbs you could also add a little tips and suggestion paper that tells the customer a bit about that particular herb and what it can be used for. You could make this on a nice light lilac colored paper with fancy print. Find a nice design for free online and print out copies of it. This will certainly add to the appeal of your clients for your products.

Marketing yourself. The best way you can market yourself is through word of mouth. Talk to your friends and neighbors telling them about your plans. You might want to consider posting flyers. Before you know it you will have your customers right in front of you waiting to purchase your wonderfully organic grown herbs!

Conclusion

I hope that my book will help guide and inspire you to delve into the world of herbal gardening, it is certainly a wonderful way to develop a business from something that you have grown passionate about as a hobby turned business. Think of all the pleasure you will find within your herbal healing garden and benefits after benefits that it will offer you for many years to come. More and more people today are seeking out organically grown plants as they are more aware of the health benefits that are attached to them. I wish you great success in building your hobby of growing herbs into a vibrant and successful business!

Thanks again for downloading my book and helping support my work. I truly do appreciate this very much indeed. I would love to read a review of my book by you on Amazon. Take care and happy herbal gardening!

FREE Bonus Reminder

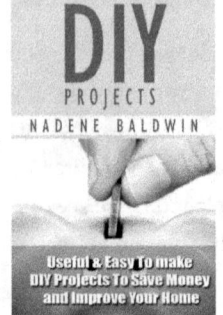

If you have not grabbed it yet, please go ahead and download your special bonus report *"DIY Projects. 13 Useful & Easy To Make DIY Projects To Save Money & Improve Your Home!"*
Simply Click the Button Below

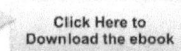

OR **Go to This Page**
http://diyhomecraft.com/free

BONUS #2: More Free & Discounted Books or Products
Do you want to receive more Free/Discounted Books or Products?
We have a mailing list where we send out our new Books or Products when they go free or with a discount on Amazon. Click on the link below to sign up for Free & Discount Book & Product Promotions.
=> Sign Up for Free & Discount Book & Product Promotions <=

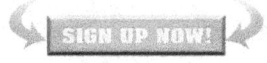

OR Go to this URL

http://zbit.ly/1WBb1Ek